Electrical Stimulation-Based Sensory Feedback in Phantom Limb Pain Treatment

Electrical Stimulation-Based Sensory Feedback in Phantom Limb Pain Treatment

PhD Thesis by

Bo Geng

Center for Sensory-Motor Interaction,
Department of Health Science and Technology,
Aalborg University, Denmark

River Publishers

Aalborg

ISBN 978-87-93102-67-5 (paperback)
ISBN 978-87-93102-42-2 (e-book)

Published, sold and distributed by:
River Publishers
Niels Jernes Vej 10
9220 Aalborg Ø
Denmark

Tel.: +45369953197
www.riverpublishers.com

Contents

Preface

The research presented in this Ph.D. thesis was carried out at the center for Sensory Motor Interaction (SMI) in the Department of Health Science and Technology of Aalborg University between 2008 and 2011. This research was financially supported by the EU-funded 'TIME' project: Transverse Intrafasicular Multichannel Electrode System, grant no. CP-FP-INFSO 224012. Completion of this thesis would not have been possible without the support of both the SMI and TIME project team.

I would like to express my sincere thanks to my supervisor, Winnie Jensen, who supported and encouraged me throughout my Ph.D. work. She gave me a chance to pursue a research topic that was new for me and provided guidance and constructive feedback. I also want to extend my thanks to Ken Yoshida for his many valuable contributions to my work. I have indeed benefited from close collaboration with him.

I would also like to thank my colleagues, who have significantly contributed to the work presented in this thesis. I would especially like to thank Laura Petrini for providing advice on psychophysical methods, Line Lindhardt Egsgaard for her help with the EEG data analysis, and Knud Larsen for his assistance in solving technical problems in the platform development. Lastly, I thank all the members of the NPI lab for the discussions on all aspects of this research, which helped shape my view on what research really is.

Special thanks go to my husband Ming for his patience and endless support and to my parents and brother, who always support me. The thesis is dedicated to our lovely daughter, Joyce, whose arrival added so much delight to my Ph.D. life.

Aalborg, June 2013

English Summary

Following amputation, up to 80% of amputees perceive pain in the missing part of the arm or leg, known as phantom limb pain (PLP). PLP can be extremely intractable, and there are no effective, long-lasting treatments currently available. Reorganization in the primary sensorimotor cortex has been found to be closely associated with PLP. Therefore, an approach targeting reversal of cortical reorganization may hold promise for PLP relief. The present thesis hypothesizes that providing sensory feedback through electrocutaneous stimulation of the residual limb may reverse cortical reorganization and consequently suppress PLP.

To address the hypothesis, five studies were conducted. Studies 1 and 2 examined the impact of stimulation parameters on the perception threshold and the evoked sensation, respectively. The stimulation location and pulse number were found to significantly affect the magnitude and quality of the perceived sensation. These two parameters were then considered to be able to effectively convey sensory information. Study 3 investigated human ability in sensory discrimination of the two identified parameters, in which satisfactory performance was obtained with able-bodied subjects. Based on the findings of the first three studies, the hypothesis was tested in study 4. An upper-limb amputee was trained in sensory identification to evaluate the effects on PLP and cortical reorganization. The results showed no changes in PLP and cortical reorganization, although the volunteer's identification accuracy improved over the course of the training period. As part of the EU-funded project 'TIME', a computerized tool was developed for evaluation of sensory feedback in a multi-channel intrafascicular stimulation system in study 5. This tool was used to assist in identifying optimal stimulation patterns that can evoke natural sensory feedback referred to the phantom limb.

Sensory feedback using direct nerve stimulation may be an alternative treatment for PLP awaiting further clinical evaluation in future work.

Danish Summary

Efter amputation føler op til 80% af de amputerede personer smerter i den manglende del af armen eller benet; dette kaldes også fantomsmerter. Fantomsmerter kan være ekstremt voldsomme og der findes ingen effektive, langvarige behandlingsmetoder mod disse smerter. Reorganisering i primær sensorisk-motorisk cortex har vist sig at være tæt forbundet med fantomsmerter. Derfor kan en metode, der er rettet imod ændring af den kortikale reorganisation vise sig at være lovende i behandlingen af fantomsmerter. Denne afhandling antager som udgangspunkt, at frembringelse af sensorisk feedback gennem elektrokutan stimulation af det resterende lem kan ændre den kortikale reorganisering og som følge heraf dæmpe fantomsmerterne.

For at underbygge denne hypotese blev der udført fem studier. Studie 1 og 2 undersøgte effekten af stimulationsparametre på henholdsvis perceptionstærsklen og den fremkaldte fornemmelse. Det blev fundet, at stimulationssted og antallet af impulser væsentligt påvirker den opfattede fornemmelses styrke og kvalitet. De to parametre blev herefter bestemt til effektivt at kunne viderebringe sensoriske informationer. Studie 3 undersøgte menneskets evne til sensorisk diskrimination af de to identificerede parametre, hvor tilfredsstillende resultater blev opnået med raske forsøgspersoner. Baseret på resultaterne af de tre første studier blev hypotesen undersøgt i studie 4. Træning af sensorisk identifikation blev undersøgt hos en person med amputation i overekstremiteten for at undersøge effekten på fantomsmerter og kortikal reorganisering. Resultaterne viste ingen ændringer i hverken fantomsmerter eller kortikal reorganisering, selvom identifikationsevnen forbedredes i træningsperioden. Som en del af det EU-finansierede projekt 'TIME' blev der i studie 5 udviklet et computerværktøj til vurdering af sensorisk feedback i et multi-kanal intrafascikulært stimulations-system. Dette blev anvendt til hjælp til identifikation af optimale stimulationsmønstre, som kan fremkalde naturlig sensorisk feedback, som refereres til fantomlemmet. Sensorisk feedback ved hjælp af direkte nervestimulation kan være en alternativ behandling for fantomsmerter, hvilket dog afventer nærmere fremtidig klinisk vurdering.

1

BACKGROUND

Surgical limb amputations are typically due to peripheral vascular diseases, cancer, or diabetes [1]. Motor vehicle accidents, wartime conflicts, terrorist attacks and landmine explosions can also necessitate traumatic limb amputation in otherwise healthy people [2]. In the USA, limb loss affects nearly 1.6 million individuals [3], and a recent study estimated that the number of people living with a limb loss will more than double by the year 2050 [4].

1.1 Non-painful phantom sensation

Virtually all amputees experience non-painful phantom sensations, i.e., the feeling that the removed limb still exists. The qualities of the phantom sensations include specific somatosensory experiences such as touch, cold, warmth, itching and other paraesthesia [5]. In addition, patients often claim they can perceive kinesthetic features, such as the size, shape, and position of the missing limb, and even voluntary movements of the phantom limb, e.g., reaching out to grab an object, making a fist or moving their fingers individually [6]. Involuntary phantom movements are also common, e.g., suddenly moving to occupy a new posture or suddenly developing a clenching spasm of the fingers [7].

Phantom sensations may be evoked by applying stimulation on the ipsilateral face or the stump (Figure 1). These phantom sensations, usually called referred sensations, i.e., sensations perceived as originating from a body site other than the one stimulated, have been described frequently following amputation [7,8,9].

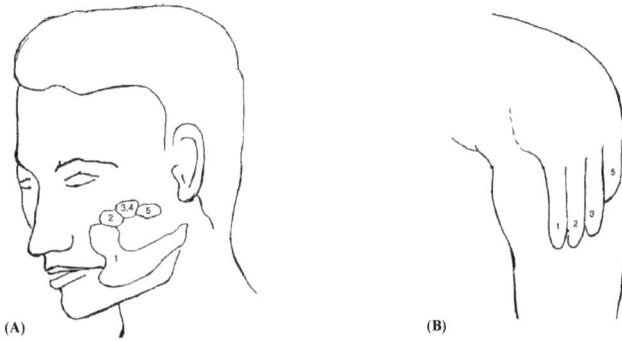

Figure 1. The distribution of referred phantom sensation in patient D. S., whose left arm was amputated 6 cm above the elbow joint due to injuries from a car accident. (A) Topographic arrangement of digits of the phantom hand on the ipsilateral face 6 months after amputation. (B) Topographic mapping of phantom digits in the region of the deltoid muscle on the stump (from Ramachandran et al. [7]).

1.2 Phantom limb pain (PLP)

1.2.1   Characteristics

In 50–85% of all amputees, pain develops in the limb that no longer exists [10]. This pain is termed phantom limb pain (PLP). PLP appears to be more common following a traumatic limb loss or if pre-amputation pain existed than after a planned surgical amputation of a non-painful limb [7]. PLP is more prevalent in adults than in children and is more prevalent in individuals who have undergone surgical amputation than in those with congenital limb deficiency [11,12]. A recent longitudinal study revealed that PLP occurs more in upper-limb than lower-limb amputees [13].

Phantom limb pain may have its onset immediately after amputation or years later [14]. In over three quarters of cases, PLP develops in the first few days following amputation [11,15,16]. PLP can persist for years and even decades. Gradual decreases in the intensity, severity, and frequency of phantom pain over time are occasionally reported [17,18,19]. However, until now there has been no evidence that the time elapsed since amputation is associated with the occurrence of PLP. Some studies have found no association between the incidence of PLP and the time since amputation [20,21]. A survey study on the long-term course of PLP in more than 500 war veterans indicated that the pain had not diminished in nearly 50% of the subjects [21]. Another large-scale survey in several thousand amputees found that more than 70% of them continued to experience PLP as much as 25 years after the amputation [22].

Most patients with PLP have intermittent pain, with intervals that range from 1 day to several weeks, while a few patients suffer constant pain. The pain often presents itself in the form of attacks that vary in duration from a few seconds to minutes or hours [23]. One in four patients experiences PLP for more than 15 hours per day [22].

The most commonly reported modalities of PLP are tingling, burning, and cramping sensations, but many other types of pain, such as throbbing, squeezing, shooting, and stabbing have also been documented [1]. The pain tends to be localized distally, regardless of the amputation site [17,18].

In approximately 50% of cases, a phenomenon called 'telescoping' occurs, i.e., the distal part of the phantom limb is progressively felt to approach the residual limb, and eventually, it may shrink within the stump [16]. Telescoping was assumed to be an adaptive process beneficial to PLP [24,25]. However, recent evidence suggests telescoping and PLP are positively related [8,26].

PLP may be elicited or worsened by a range of physical factors (e.g., weather change or pressure on the residual limb) or psychological factors (e.g., emotional stress) [27,28]. Cognitive factors also play a part in the modulation of PLP. Patients who have personality traits characterized by passive coping are more affected by the pain and report more interference [29].

In summary, PLP can be extremely intractable and disabling. It is sufficiently severe to hamper prosthetic training [30] and reduce amputees' likelihood of employment and social activities [31]. Apart from its negative impacts on patients' functioning and well-being [32,33], PLP also poses a significant problem for health care systems worldwide [34]. Thus, successful intervention for treatment of PLP is greatly needed.

1.2.2   Neurobiological mechanisms

PLP is usually classified as neuropathic pain, which involves multiple pathophysiological changes, both in the peripheral nervous system (PNS) and in the central nervous system (CNS) [35,36,37]. After surgical removal of a limb, the complete truncation of peripheral nerves and the neural damage initiate a cascade of changes that lead to and sustain phantom pain, which might be the manifestation of maladaptive plasticity in the nervous system [38]. No single mechanism appears to be able to explain the development of PLP independently. Hence, it is currently believed that PLP should be considered a complex syndrome and that multiple mechanisms at different levels in the nervous system contribute to the occurrence of PLP.

Peripheral mechanisms

Following truncation of peripheral nerves, a neuroma is universally formed as a result of aberrant sprouting of regenerating axons. Ectopic discharge from a stump neuroma has been postulated as one important peripheral mechanism. Such neuromas show spontaneous discharge or hyper-excitability following mechanical and chemical stimulation [39]. In addition, similar abnormal activity and sensitivity occurs in dorsal root ganglia (DRG), where the discharge coming from the residual limb can be amplified (Devor, Seltzer, 1999). In addition, abnormal sympathetic activity may increase the amount of circulating epinephrine, which can trigger and exacerbate neuronal activity from neuroma [40]. These aberrant nociceptive impulses may be interpreted by the brain as pain.

One of the strongest arguments for a peripheral cause of phantom limb pain is its positive correlation with stump pain. Phantom pain occurs significantly more frequently in amputees with chronic stump pain than in those without stump pain [41]. Nevertheless, peripheral factors alone cannot entirely explain the occurrence of PLP. In some cases, PLP occurs immediately after amputation when there are not yet neuromas in the residual limb

[42]. Congenital amputees occasionally also report PLP [12]. These findings indicate that central factors must be involved as well.

Central mechanisms

While spinal plasticity (e.g., sensitization of low-threshold sensory receptors and central sensitization [36,43]) have been discussed as processes involved in PLP or neuropathic pain, cortical plasticity or cortical reorganization has gained a great deal of attention and is considered a plausible explanation for PLP. Furthermore, cortical reorganization may partly account for why stimulation on the face, stump or surrounding regions elicit sensations referred to the phantom limb [44].

Extensive empirical studies have demonstrated that sensorimotor cortices undergo massive neuroplasticity changes in people with extremity amputation [20,45,46,47]. The cortical area that formerly represented the amputated extremity has been found to be taken over by its neighboring mouth and chin representation zone in the primary somatosensory cortex (S1) of amputees [48,49]. Further studies have found that cortical reorganization also develops in the motor cortex (M1) [50,51,52].

Furthermore, the extent of cortical reorganization has been found to be closely associated with the severity of phantom pain and the size of the deafferented region. A series of studies have revealed a positive relation between the magnitude of PLP and the amount of reorganization in the sensorimotor cortices [50,51,52,53]. Cortical remapping may be related to the incongruence of motor intentions and sensory feedback, based on maladaptive plastic changes in the brain [54].

Neuroplasticity has also been observed in the thalamus and has shown close relation to the perception of phantom limbs and phantom pain, according to the results of thalamic stimulation and recordings in human amputees [55]. Experiments in monkeys have shown that the changes can be relayed from the spinal and brainstem level [56], but those on the subcortical levels may also originate in the cortex, which has strong efferent connections to the thalamus and lower structures [57].

1.2.3   State-of-the-art treatments for phantom limb pain

Commonly used treatments for PLP can be categorized as pharmacological, surgical, anesthetic, psychological, or other methods [35]. The following is a brief description of each category.

Pharmacological

Numerous pharmacological interventions have been reported, such as N-methyl D-aspartate receptor antagonists, antidepressants, anticonvulsants, neuroleptics, β-blockers, and muscle relaxants [23,58]. Despite many drugs or combination of drugs tried over decades, mixed results have been obtained, with some studies showing positive outcomes and others showing no efficacy [58].

Surgical

Conventional surgical methods include stump revision, neurectomy, rhizotomy, cordotomy sympathectomy, tractotomy etc [35]. In general, these treatments have shown unfavorable results for decades and have been most abandoned, as the surgical procedures may carry a risk of further nerve damage [1].

Neurostimulation based on surgery is also grouped in this category. Deep brain stimulation (DBS) of the periventricular grey (PVG) and sensory thalamus has shown promise as an effective treatment for peripheral neuropathic pain and PLP [59,60]. Relief of PLP has also been achieved by spinal cord stimulation (SCS) and motor cortex stimulation (MCS) [61,62]. While neurostimulation appears to be promising, it is currently difficult to assess its effectiveness because of the lack of long-term controlled studies.

Anesthetic

Many studies have examined the effectiveness of epidural anesthesia but unfortunately have not been consistent in their experimental designs and have yielded inconsistent results [63,64]. Other anesthetic methods, including nerve blocks, sympathetic blocks, and local anesthesia, have also been used, while no well-controlled studies have demonstrated long-lasting favorable effects on diminishing PLP.

Psychological

Several studies have suggested that temperature and electromyography (EMG) biofeedback may be helpful in alleviating burning and cramping PLP sensations [65,66]. However, there is no evidence to match specific types of phantom pain with specific biofeedback techniques [67]. Hypnosis has also been anecdotally reported as being effective in PLP relief [68].

Other approaches

Transcutaneous electrical nerve stimulation (TENS) has been recommended as a treatment option for phantom pain and stump pain [69]. In multiple placebo-controlled trials and epidemiologic surveys [21,43,70], desensitization resulting from TENS application has been reported to be capable of relieving PLP. However, its long-term effectiveness remains unclear. Some studies have suggested that PLP reductions after 1 year of TENS treatment are comparable to those achieved using placebos [71].

Mirror therapy appears to be a promising treatment option. In mirror therapy, patients are given the visual illusion that they can use their missing limbs again [72,73]. Recently, a randomized, sham-controlled, crossover study of mirror therapy indicated that it achieved a significant decrease in pain intensity, whereas two control groups did not show satisfactory treatment outcomes [73]. Despite the success of this therapy, the underlying mechanism accounting for the success remains to be elucidated, and more experiments are needed to replicate the results.

Many other treatments for PLP, such vibration, acupuncture, mental imagery, ultrasound, massage, electroconvulsive therapy, electromagnetic fields, and far infrared rays, have been reported in small-sample-size studies and case reports [69,74,75,76,77,78,79]. Although many therapies for PLP have been attempted or are currently in use, most appear ineffective or limited in their effectiveness. It is thus critical to develop effective treatments for PLP.

1.3 Sensory feedback

1.3.1   Sensory feedback for PLP treatment

Behaviorally relevant interventions that provide feedback to the brain may modify the cortical mapping in brain areas such as the primary somatosensory cortex (S1). In the adult owl monkey, several weeks of tactile discrimination training of individual fingers led to an expansion of the cortices representing the trained fingers in the S1 zone, whereas cortical alteration was not observed after passive stimulation [80]. Change in the topographic organization of the hand representation zone was also observed after training in a frequency discrimination task [81].

Phantom limb pain has been found to be related to reorganization in S1. There is a significant correlation between the severity of PLP and the amount of cortical reorganization [8,82]. It therefore has been postulated that interventions designed to reverse somatosensory cortical reorganization may be valuable alternative treatments for PLP and neuropathic pain [83]. Providing cognitive behavior-relevant sensory feedback may be able to address the incongruence between motor intention and sensory feedback and consequently relieve phantom pain through normalization of cortical somatosensory representation maps.

Several studies have demonstrated the beneficial effect of enhancing somatosensory feedback on PLP and cortical reorganization. In a study on the effect of sensory discrimination training on PLP, amputee patients were asked to perform the task of discriminating among the locations and frequencies of the surface electrical stimuli applied to the residual limb. After two weeks of daily training, all five patients in the training group experienced significant decreases in PLP, compared with a control group that received regular treatments. Their discrimination ability was also improved, and the amount of cortical reorganization was reduced

[84]. In another study, intensive use of myoelectric prosthesis led to significant reduction in PLP [85]. It has also been reported that training for control of a robotic hand with a limited amount of sensory feedback significantly reduced PLP in a human amputee implanted with four intra-fascicular electrodes in the nerve stump. The reduction in PLP lasted several weeks after removal of the electrodes, and changes in sensorimotor cortex topography were observed [86]. A recent study found that usage of a prosthesis that provides somatosensory feedback on the grip strength was effective in alleviating PLP [87]. Furthermore, tactile discrimination, rather than passive stimulation, relieved pain and improved tactile acuity in patients with chronic pain [88]. These findings suggest the therapeutic benefit of somatosensory feedback in the treatment of PLP and chronic pain.

1.3.2   Means of providing sensory feedback

Although sensory feedback has been proposed for the treatment of PLP, it was first recognized as being greatly needed for better control of prosthetic devices and improving body awareness of artificial limbs. Artificial sensory feedback is intended to provide users who have lost their sensory functions with regained tactile and kinesthetic sensibilities. For decades, the development of artificial sensory inputs to a sensory feedback system for prostheses has been mainly based on mechanical stimulation, electrocutaneous stimulation, and direct nerve stimulation.

Mechanical stimulation

Mechanical stimulation, which can be applied in two ways, by vibration or by static pressure, conveys sensory information by activation of mechanoreceptors in the skin using an actuator [89]. Mechanical sensory feedback systems generally have higher universal psychological acceptance than electrocutaneous systems because the vibration and pressure sensation feel more natural. While mechanical transducers have occasionally been criticized as being bulky, heavy, moving, and power-consuming, a comparative study suggested that it is capable of yielding performance comparable to electrocutaneous stimulation [90]. In several studies, different types of small, low-power motors were evaluated successfully for application in shoulder pad displays [91] and sensory feedback in prosthetic systems [92,93].

Electrocutaneous stimulation

In electrocutaneous stimulation, electrical current flows through the skin and evokes sensations by directly activating afferent nerve fibers [94]. It has also been suggested that small electrodes (1 mm^2) activate receptors or end organs in the dermis [95]. Subjects describe the qualities of the sensations evoked by electrocutaneous stimulation as tingles, itches, vibrations, buzzes, touches, pressure, pinches, and sharp and burning pain. The sensations originate in the skin but are not necessarily confined to a small region of skin when deeper nerve bundles are stimulated. The sensation evoked is a function of many factors, including the stimulating voltage, the current, the waveform, the electrode size, the material, the location on the skin, the thickness, and the degree of hydration [89].

    The use of electrocutaneous stimulation to generate sensory feedback has attracted great attention because of its ability to provide densely packed information and produce a sensation whose frequency and intensity can be reliably controlled [94]. Unlike mechanical vibrators, cutaneous electrodes usually have no moving parts and maintain constant contact with the skin. In addition, they are efficient in terms of power consumption and are simple to fabricate [94]. A series of studies have shown that sensory feedback employing electrocutaneous stimulation improves the level of a subject's confidence in using a hand prosthesis and facilitates the incorporation of the prosthesis into body image [96,97,98,99,100].

Intra-neural stimulation

When electrical stimulation is applied directly to the nerve in a residual limb, possible activation of small clusters of sensory neurons at a subfascicular level may evoke more natural, meaningful sensations. This was demonstrated in a study in human amputees with micro-fabricated longitudinal intra-fascicular electrodes (LIFE) implanted in their median/ulnar nerve stumps. The stimulations generated discrete, graded sensations of touch/pressure, joint position or movement of the phantom hand, although the proprioceptive perceptions were reported to be vague, and the interpretation was therefore difficult [101]. A recent study used newer-generation, thin-film LIFEs with more stimulating channels implanted in the median/ulnar nerves of an amputee volunteer for four weeks. The results showed that during the initial experiments, the patient reported various sensations after stimulation at low to moderate levels, although tactile sensations could only be generated within the first 10 days [86]. Although many problems, including development of biochemically resistant electrodes with high selectivity and evaluation of long-term effects, remain to be investigated, intra-neural stimulation might be another viable means of artificially providing sensory feedback in the future.

1.3.3   Measurement of sensory feedback

Cutaneous sensory feedback is essentially the transmission of sensory information from the skin to the brain. Electrocutaneous stimulation activates sensory neurons in or under the skin. Neural signals passing via sensory nerves to the brain evoke subjective experience of the stimulus and produce a sensation. Psychophysical methods can be used to quantitatively investigate the relation between electrical stimuli and subjective sensations [102].

Measurement of the perception threshold is usually the first step in design of a sensory feedback scheme because the stimulus current amplitude between the perception threshold and the upper limit should be carefully determined. Since the perception threshold is a function of the electric charge in the context of electrocutaneous stimulation, a lower threshold is preferred for its better energy efficiency [94]. Among the three classical psychophysical methods for perception threshold measurement (i.e., the method of adjustment, the method of limits, and the method of constant stimuli), the method of constant stimuli is generally considered to provide the most reliable estimate of the threshold because a random presentation of stimuli can efficiently eliminate possible bias from a subject's anticipation [103].

In a sensory feedback scheme, evoked sensation ideally should be strong but without discomfort. Measurement of a sensation involves evaluation of the sensation quality (or type) and estimation of the sensation intensity.

The qualities of the sensations evoked by cutaneous electrical stimulation have been documented in the literature mainly in the forms of descriptive words reported by subjects, such as touch, pressure, tingling, and vibration. As a general rule in psychophysics, questions that are precise and simple enough to obtain convincing answer should be formulated [103]. Thus, a question that provides subjects with a group of descriptors covering possibly elicited sensation types may be used to evaluate the quality of sensation.

The intensity of sensation can be quantitatively estimated using a scaling method by assigning numbers to the perceptual event such as sensation [104]. A visual analogue scale (VAS) can be used to measure a sensation, with 0 representing 'no sensation' and 10 representing 'the upper limit of the sensation or pain.' There are also a number of other types of linear scales, such as the Likert scale and the Borg scale, which may outperform others in specific circumstances [105].

1.4 The EU TIME project

Part of this PhD research was involved in the EU consortium's TIME project. The goal of the TIME project was to develop an implantable neural prosthesis system with sufficient stimulation selectivity to manipulate phantom sensations and explore the possibility of using the method as a potentially effective treatment for PLP. Given sufficient control over a large set of afferent fibers and fiber types, stimulation via a neural interface is able to artificially evoke sensations of touch, vibration, heat, and illusions of limb/ finger/joint position and movement. In the case of amputees, precise activation of the intact part of the transacted sensory fibers through a selective multi-channel electrode may elicit vivid sensations in the phantom limb. The TIME project hypothesizes that manipulating phantom sensations using selective stimulation of the nerve stump may mitigate PLP and reverse cortical reorganization. The hypothesis is illustrated in Figure 3.

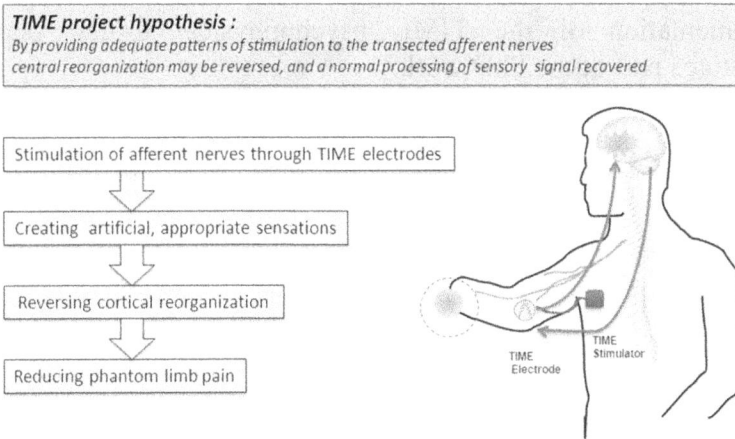

Figure 2. Illustration of the hypothesis in the TIME project.

The TIME project consists of three core technological challenges: (1) development of a novel micro-fabricated neural interface—the Thin-film Intrafascicular Multichannel Electrode array (TIME)—to be implanted in the nerve stump, (2) development of a human-implantable multichannel stimulator system, and (3) development of a psychophysical testing platform that can support effective and efficient evaluation of phantom sensations evoked by multi-channel selective micro-stimulation.

Because the optimal set of stimulation patterns that can generate natural phantom sensations has not been well identified in the literature, various combinations of stimulation parameters were considered. A TIME electrode array features up to 12 active contact sites [106]. Different combinations of stimulus parameters in the TIME multichannel system can result in a wide range of possible stimulation patterns. In a clinical trial, to reduce a patient's mental load and avoid habituation to the stimulation, it is important to test a large number of stimuli efficiently within a limited experiment time. Therefore, an automated stimulation and evaluation process is necessary to minimize the time needed to collect the measurement data from the patient. A computerized platform can support the automated process of stimulation and evaluation. Design and implementation of the TIME psychophysical testing platform constitutes part of the PhD work.

2

OVERVIEW OF THE PHD WORK

2.1 Hypothesis and research questions

As stated in the previous section, the severity of PLP was found to be positively associated with the amount of cortical alteration [8]. Because cortical changes in the brain may result from the incongruence of motor intention and impaired sensory feedback due to transection of periphery nerves [54], artificially providing adequate feedback of the phantom limb may assist in addressing the incongruence. The scientific hypothesis of the present PhD research was the following:

> *Providing sensory feedback through electrocutaneous stimulation of a residual limb may reverse cortical alteration and consequently reduce PLP.*

To test the hypothesis, three questions were formulated:

- *Question 1. How do stimulus parameters influence sensory responses?*
- *Question 2. Does sensory identification training have a therapeutic benefit for PLP?*
- *Question 3. How may sensory feedback be evaluated efficiently in a multi-channel stimulation setting?*

The sensation elicited by electrocutaneous stimulation is a function of the stimulation parameters. The stimulus parameters selected to be modulated to convey sensory information play important roles in determining the effectiveness of a sensory feedback scheme. It is thus important to examine how stimulus parameters influence sensory responses (Question 1). Furthermore, training patients in discriminating among different stimulus parameters has been proven to have a positive effect on PLP [84]. Sensory identification is a moderately more complex behaviorally relevant task that is assumed to involve more sophisticated sensory processing. Does sensory identification training have a therapeutic benefit for PLP (Question 2)? Given the multichannel, intra-neural stimulation system developed in the TIME project, how may sensory feedback be evaluated effectively and efficiently (Question 3)?

Electrocutaneous stimulation, rather than mechanical stimulation, was chosen as the means of delivering sensory feedback, mainly for the following reasons: (1) it is likely to produce more types of sensation, which may involve more sensory processing and thus act on the sensory cortices more effectively; (2) stimulation parameters are more controllable, which partly ensures the reliability of the sensory feedback; and (3) many product options for electrodes are commercially available.

2.2 Studies and scientific papers

To address the three questions raised, five studies were conducted in this PhD research. Question 1 was addressed through examination of the impact of stimulation parameters on the perception threshold in Study 1 and the impact on evoked sensation magnitude, quality, and location in Study 2. Question 2 was addressed in Studies 3 and 4. Study 3 investigated human ability to identify the stimulation location and pulse number in behaviorally relevant tasks with able-bodied subjects. In study 4, an upper-limb amputee volunteer with PLP was trained in sensory identification to examine the effect of training on identification performance, the intensity of PLP, and cortical reorganization. Question 3 was addressed by design and development of a computerized, automated psychophysical test platform in Study 5. An overview of the objectives, subjects, and methodologies of the five specific studies is presented in Table 1.

Table 1. Overview of the five studies conducted in this PhD research, including objectives, subjects, and methodologies.

Study	Objective	Subject	Methodology
Study 1	Investigation of the impact of selected stimulation parameters on the perception threshold	12 able-bodied	**Electrodes**: 5 solid-gel Ag/AgCl electrodes. **Placement**: 5 cm from the elbow crease, evenly distributed around the left forearm. **Measure**: Perception threshold **Investigated parameters**: location, number of active electrodes, number of pulses, and interleaved time between a pair of electrodes.
Study 2	Evaluation of the impact of selected stimulation parameters on evoked sensations	16 able-bodied	**Electrodes and Placement**: same as study 1. **Measure**: sensation modality, location, quality, and magnitude **Investigated parameters**: same as study 1
Study 3	Examination of the sensory identification ability of able-bodied subjects	10 able-bodied	**Electrodes**: 3 solid-gel Ag/AgCl electrodes. **Placement**: 5 cm from the elbow crease, on the volar side of the left forearm. **Measure**: identification performance **Tasks**: Identification among 5 stimulation locations, 5 pulse numbers, 10 paired combinations of stimulation location and pulse number.
Study 4	Exploration of the effect of sensory identification training on PLP and cortical reorganization	1 upper-limb amputee	**Electrodes**: 8 solid-gel Ag/AgCl electrodes **Placement**: on the stump such that the evoked sensations referred to different locations in the phantom hand. **Treatment**: daily 1-hr training consisted of three sessions in which the subject was asked to identify: A) stimulating site, B) number of pulses (1, 2, 5, 10, and 20), C) combination of location and pulse number. **Measure**: PLP (VAS), identification accuracy, and cortical plasticity (hd-EEG).
Study 5	Design and development of a computerized tool to control and evaluate multi-channel electrical stimulation-based sensory feedback	NA	**Functionalities:** A) Configuration of stimuli, control of experiment, and monitoring experimental progress. B) Threshold measure, sensation measure, and collection of the measurement data, and C) Communication between SEC and ISI to achieve the automated process of stimulation and sensation evaluation.

Study 1

Published in: Journal of Neuroengineering Rehabilitation 2011, 8:9.
Impacts of selected stimulation patterns on the perception threshold in electrocutaneous stimulation

Bo Geng[1], Ken Yoshida[2], Winnie Jensen[1]

[1]Center for Sensory-Motor Interaction, Dept. Health Science and Technology, Aalborg University, Denmark; [2]Biomedical Engineering Department, Indiana University-Purdue University Indianapolis, Indianapolis, USA

Corresponding author:
Bo Geng
Center for Sensory-motor Interaction
Department of Health Science and Technology, Aalborg University
Fredrik Bajersvej 7D, 9220 Aalborg, Denmark
bogeng@hst.aau.dk

Study 2

Published in: Journal of Rehabilitation Research and Development 2012, 49(2): 297-308.

Evaluation of sensation evoked by electrocutaneous stimulation on forearm in nondisabled subjects

Bo Geng[1], Ken Yoshida[2], Laura Petrini[1, 3], Winnie Jensen[1]

[1]Center for Sensory-Motor Interaction, Dept. Health Science and Technology, Aalborg University, Denmark; [2]Biomedical Engineering Department, Indiana University-Purdue University Indianapolis, Indianapolis, USA; [3]Department of Communication and Psychology, Aalborg University, Denmark

Corresponding author:
Bo Geng
Center for Sensory-motor Interaction
Department of Health Science and Technology, Aalborg University
Fredrik Bajersvej 7D, 9220 Aalborg, Denmark
bogeng@hst.aau.dk

Study 3

Submitted to Journal of Neuroengineering and Rehabilitation.
Human ability in identification of location and pulse number for electrocutaneous stimulation applied on the forearm

Bo Geng[1], Winnie Jensen[1]

[1]Center for Sensory-Motor Interaction, Dept. Health Science and Technology, Aalborg University, Denmark

Corresponding author:
Bo Geng
Center for Sensory-motor Interaction
Department of Health Science and Technology, Aalborg University
Fredrik Bajersvej 7D, 9220 Aalborg, Denmark
bogeng@hst.aau.dk

Study 4

Published in Annual meeting of Society for Neuroscience, Neuroscience 2011.
A case study on phantom sensation and sensory discrimination induced by electrocutaneous stimulation

Bo Geng[1], Ken Yoshida[2], Winnie Jensen[1]

[1] Center for Sensory-Motor Interaction, Dept. Health Science and Technology, Aalborg University, Denmark; [2] Biomedical Engineering Department, Indiana University-Purdue University Indianapolis, Indianapolis, USA

Corresponding author:
Bo Geng
Center for Sensory-motor Interaction
Department of Health Science and Technology, Aalborg University
Fredrik Bajersvej 7D, 9220 Aalborg, Denmark
bogeng@hst.aau.dk

Study 5

Computerized tool to control and evaluate multi-channel electrical stimulation based sensory feedback—example of use for phantom limb pain treatment
Bo Geng[1], Ken Yoshida[2], Winnie Jensen[1]

[1]Center for Sensory-Motor Interaction, Dept. Health Science and Technology, Aalborg University, Denmark; [2]Biomedical Engineering Department, Indiana University-Purdue University Indianapolis, Indianapolis, USA;

Corresponding author:
Bo Geng
Center for Sensory-motor Interaction
Department of Health Science and Technology, Aalborg University
Fredrik Bajersvej 7D, 9220 Aalborg, Denmark
bogeng@hst.aau.dk

3

DISCUSSION AND CONCLUSIONS

Five studies were performed to address the hypothesis and the three formulated questions. The main outcomes and related issues of the Ph.D. research have been discussed here, whereas a more detailed discussion of specific studies can be found in relevant papers. Some perspectives pertaining to this research topic are also discussed, as appropriate.

3.1 Discussion of the main findings

An overview of the main findings of each study is outlined in Table 2. In summary, the ventral forearm had a lower perception threshold than the dorsal forearm. The stimulation location on the forearm significantly influenced the sensory responses. The number of pulses also had a significant impact on the perceived magnitude of sensation. When the stimulation location and pulse number were varied in identification tasks, satisfactory identification performance was achieved by able-bodied subjects. However, training in the same sensory identification tasks neither relieved PLP nor reversed cortical reorganization in the amputee patient, although the amputee patient's identification performance improved over the training period. In addition, a computerized sensory feedback evaluation platform developed for the TIME project made a tool for further studies on PLP treatment by providing patients with more intuitive, natural sensory feedback using selective intra-neural stimulation. Each study is discussed below in relation to the three questions.

Table 2. Major outcomes of each study.

Overall hypothesis: *Providing sensory feedback through electrocutaneous stimulation of a residual limb may reverse cortical alteration and consequently reduce PLP.*			
	Q1: How do stimulation parameters influence sensory input?	*Q2: Does sensory identification training have therapeutic benefit for PLP?*	*Q3: How may sensory feedback be evaluated efficiently in a multi-channel stimulation setting?*
Study 1: Impact of selected stimulation parameters on perception threshold	(1) Ventral forearm has a lower perception threshold than the dorsal side. (2) Perception threshold reversely related to the pulse number.		
Study 2: Impact of selected stimulation parameters on evoked sensations	(1)Volar and ulnar forearm perceived touch sensation more consistently. (2) The pulse number significantly influences the perceived intensity.		
Study 3: Sensory identification ability of able-bodied subjects		Average performance in identification of stimulation location and pulse number was promising.	
Study 4: Effect of sensory identification training on PLP and cortical plasticity		Identification accuracy improved, but without cortical changes and PLP.	
Study 5: A tool to control and evaluate multi-channel electrical stimulation-based sensory feedback			The tool was used for threshold and sensation measurement in the clinical experiments with an amputee volunteer.

Study 1: Effect of stimulation parameters on the perception threshold (Q1)

By examining the relation between stimulation parameters and the perception threshold, study 1 provided useful information for optimization of a stimulation protocol in a sensory feedback scheme. The ventral aspect of the forearm was found to have a lower perception threshold than the dorsal aspect. Therefore, use of the ventral forearm is recommended for receiving electrocutaneous sensory feedback, due to the better energy efficiency and potentially higher information transfer capacity that it provides.

Sensory feedback should be consistent to gain users' confidence in interpreting artificial sensory input. However, consistency cannot be guaranteed because of the non-linear relation between the stimulation parameters and sensory responses [95]. This is confirmed by the results of study 1. The four parameters investigated—stimulation location, number of stimulating channels, number of pulses, and time delay in interleaved stimulation—were all shown to be related to the perception threshold in a non-linear way.

The stimulation parameters investigated were chosen on the basis of a literature review and the need for sensory feedback in amputee patients. Some parameters, such as body locus, pulse duration, waveform, and frequency, have been investigated in previous studies [107,108,109]. Those studies mainly concerned single-channel stimulation using different types of surface electrodes at various body sites, whereas study 1 investigated the parameters in relation to multi-channel stimulation on the forearm with solid-gel electrodes.

Study 2: Effect of stimulation parameters on evoked sensation (Q1)

Study 2 provided information used in the choice of the optimal stimulation parameters to be used for sensory modulation. Varying a stimulation parameter can modulate the sensation by which information is encoded and transmitted to human subjects [94]. If the sensation (e.g., intensity or modality) can be easily and reliably modulated by varying a stimulation parameter, the coding scheme was assumed to be effective.

In study 2, stimulation of the ventral forearm was found to more easily evoke tactile and less pricking sensation than stimulation of the dorsal side. This finding is important to ensure the comfort of electrocutaneous sensory feedback, as electrical stimulation is often associated with discomfort and occasionally pain, which can be a limiting factor in users' acceptance [110,111]. Other elements, such as electrode size, waveform, and frequency, may also have an impact on the comfort of electrocutaneous stimulation [112,113,114].

Furthermore, the number of pulses has a significant effect on the perceived magnitude, implying that varying the number of pulses may be an effective means of sensory modulation. This finding is consistent with those of a recent study [115]. An early study derived a specific relation for pulse number growing as the 1.8 power of the perceived magnitude in stimulation applied on the abdomen at 30 Hz [116].

Study 3: Sensory identification in able-bodied subjects (Q2)

In study 3, the sensory identification ability of able-bodied subjects was evaluated. Based on the findings of studies 1 and 2, electrodes were placed on the ventral forearm. The stimulation location and pulse number were varied for purposes of sensory modulation.

Modulation of the two parameters yielded satisfactory identification performance. The overall accuracy was 92.2% for spatial identification and 90.8% for the identification of the pulse number. Performance worsened when the two dimensions were required to be distinguished at the same time. The results provide an opportunity to directly compare the identification performance of able-bodied subjects and amputees, which can assist in translating the findings to clinical application. However, to the best of my knowledge, there have been no such studies on sensory identification with upper-limb amputees. The only related work has been on the effect of sensory discrimination training on PLP. In that study, amputee subjects were trained in sensory discrimination of stimulation location and frequency. Discriminability was shown to be improved over the two weeks of the training period, but the accuracy remained below 60% for both location and frequency discrimination [84].

Study 4: Sensory feedback training in amputee patients (Q2)

In study 4, an amputee patient was trained in sensory identification to investigate the effect of training on PLP. The stimulation location and pulse number were again varied for purposes of sensory modulation. It was expected that the identification ability of amputees would be better than that of able-bodied subjects because stimulation of the residual limb can evoke sensations not only locally but also referred to the phantom limb [45], implying that the somatosensory cortex representing the forearm may be expanded and thus that sensory acuity may be improved in amputees. However, the amputee patient did not achieve good identification performance in the first days of training. Over the training period, the amputee patient's accuracy improved and was eventually comparable to that of the able-bodied subjects. The unexpected low identification ability of the amputee patient at the beginning of the training period was likely due to subject-to-subject variance in learning rates. Research into the identification abilities of more amputees is needed to allow for statistical comparison between the two groups.

No reduction in PLP and no changes in cortical reorganization were observed after ten days of training. Nevertheless, the failure of sensory identification training in PLP treatment should be interpreted with caution. First of all, the training might not have been extensive enough, or the stimulus intensity might not have been sufficiently strong. A similar study on the effect of feedback-guided sensory training on PLP was performed with ten daily 90-min training sessions and a stimulus level of 0.1 mA below the individual pain threshold [84]. In that study, all five amputee patients experienced reductions in PLP and reversal of cortical reorganization. A comparative study is needed to validate the training regimen. Furthermore, cortical reorganization alone might not be the primary factor in the development of PLP in this patient. Providing sensory feedback of the phantom hand with the aim of counteracting cortical reorganization might thus be ineffective for him. This may further confirm that various mechanisms account for the causation and maintenance of PLP in individual patients and that no one treatment is likely to be effective for all amputee patients [35]. Appropriate selection of interventions that can address the underlying problems will be important for effective PLP treatment.

A follow-up study with a larger sample size and perhaps a higher stimulation intensity is needed to further evaluate the effect of sensory identification training on PLP. Additionally, in what subgroup of amputee patients, sensory feedback-based intervention is effective remains to be investigated. To what extent the number of training sessions and the stimulus intensity would affect the treatment outcome also needs to be determined.

Study 5: Computerized psychophysical testing platform (Q3)

Recently, peripheral intra-neural interfaces with multiple channels have been developed for direct nerve stimulation with high selectivity, which could be used to record motor signals in bionic hand control [86,106,117]. Using the same electrodes to selectively activate sensory fibers in the nerve bundle provides the possibility to manipulate phantom sensation [117] and counteract phantom pain by enabling sensory processing that is missing subsequent to amputation.

To efficiently evaluate the phantom sensation evoked by a wide range of stimulation patterns in a multi-channel setting, a computerized psychophysical testing platform was developed. The platform was designed to collect the data from the threshold and sensation measure experiments. However, to counteract cortical alterations and consequently relieve PLP, it was expected that repeated stimulation sessions with one subject would need to be carried out. Hence, selection of a subset of optimal stimulation patterns was required for each subject, based on the results of the sensation measurements. Optimal stimulation patterns were defined as those that elicited clear, distinct types of sensations referred to the phantom limb. Therefore, a module that can automatically select optimal stimulation patterns should be considered in future development.

3.2 Methodological considerations

Studies with able-bodied subjects

The first three studies were conducted with able-bodied subjects. It is noteworthy that the sample population is not representative of amputee patients with PLP. Therefore, the results ought to be carefully interpreted before implementation in amputee patients, because when stimulating damaged limbs, the perceptual experience may differ from those in nondisabled people. It will be of interest to see whether similar results can be obtained with subjects with amputations in future work.

Choice of stimulation parameters

Throughout studies 1 to 4, a biphasic waveform was used because the dermis accumulates electrochemical changes from monophasic pulses. In addition, biphasic pulse pairs produce less long-term reddening and a more comfortable sensation than monophasic pulses [94]. A pulse duration of 200 µs was chosen because it produced the least 'pricking' sensation in our pilot experiment, in which pulse durations of 100 µs, 200 µs and 500 µs were tested. A frequency of 20 Hz was used because this may be the optimal frequency for sensory communication, as the maximum frequency discrimination occurs near 20 Hz [118].

Stimulation parameters related to dual channel stimulation were investigated in studies 1 and 2 because incorporation of a second channel introduces additional variables that can affect the efficacy of sensory feedback [94]. As a limitation, only a selected set of stimulation parameters (i.e., the stimulation site, the number of stimulating channels, the number of pulses, and the time delay between two channels) were examined in studies 1 and 2.

Sensory identification

Both animal and human experiments have revealed that training in sensory discrimination, rather than passive stimulation, can result in cortical remodeling [81,84]. In discrimination tasks, a subject needs to determine whether there is a detectable difference between the presented stimulus and the reference stimulus. In identification tasks, the subject needs to identify the presented stimulus among several different stimuli. Sensory identification requires not only detecting the difference between two stimuli presented but also determining which stimulus was presented. As such, it is assumed that sensory identification involves more advanced cognitive activity, such as attention and memory, than does sensory discrimination or passive stimulation and consequently facilitates cortex remapping. This assumption led to studies 3 and 4, in which sensory identification was chosen as the means of providing sensory feedback to the subjects.

Measurement of cortical reorganization

In the study 4 on the effect of sensory identification training on PLP, cortical reorganization was assessed before and after training. Neuroelectrical source analysis of high-density EEG recording was used to localize the cortical activity. Light superficial pressure stimulation was applied to the corner of the lower lip because the cortical area representing the mouth was found to take over the former hand area [45,48]. The patient's phantom pain and the observation of the shift of the lip area to the hand area on the amputation side confirmed the earlier proposed theory that cortical reorganization is related to PLP [8,84,119].

However, the PLP was not reduced after the sensory identification training, and the cortical shift was not reversed. From the perspective of the technology employed, although EEG source analysis is occasionally used to localize brain activity, it suffers from the limitation of poor spatial resolution. The accuracy of EEG source analysis is affected by many practical factors, such as the electrode position on the scalp, the choice of reference, the interpolation algorithm chosen, the treatment of artifact-contaminated channels due to poor electrode–scalp contact or amplifier malfunction, and the head model and mathematical inverse model chosen [120]. In this regard, other imaging methods, such as fMRI, might be better suited to localization of brain activity and ensure the validity of the results.

Electrocutaneous vs. intra-neural sensory feedback

Sensory feedback employing electrocutaneous stimulation has been shown to be somewhat successful in PLP treatment [84,87]. Its noninvasiveness is also attractive. However, electrocutaneous stimulation can only elicit somatic sensation (e.g., touch, tingling) locally or in the phantom limb, which greatly limits the utilization of sensory feedback. Performing behaviorally relevant discrimination and identification tasks is then used as an alternative means of providing meaningful sensory feedback. Incorporation of other sensory modality feedback (e.g., visual, audio) may enhance its effectiveness in counteracting the cortical reorganization underlying PLP.

Direct nerve stimulation made it possible to evoke more types of meaningful sensory feedback (e.g., finger movement, joint position, wrist movement) [101]. Moreover, it has the advantage of using the same set of implanted electrodes for both bionic hand control and sensory feedback. In particular, the patient who participated in study 4 was later treated by providing sensory feedback using intrafascicular stimulation with implanted TIME electrodes, and PLP was temporarily alleviated within the implantation period (results not published). This is an exciting clue that encourages further exploration of this type of sensory feedback in PLP treatment.

3.3 Conclusions

This PhD thesis has presented five studies to address the hypothesis that providing sensory feedback through electrocutaneous stimulation of a residual limb may reverse cortical alteration and consequently reduce PLP in amputee patients. The impact of stimulation parameters on the perception threshold and the evoked sensation was examined. The stimulation location and pulse number were identified to be able to effectively convey sensory information. Human ability in sensory identification of the two parameters was then investigated, and satisfactory performance was obtained in able-bodied subjects. On the basis of these findings, the hypothesis was tested by providing sensory identification training to an upper-limb amputee volunteer. However, PLP and cortical reorganization in this patient did not show significant changes. Direct afferent nerve stimulation of the residual limb makes it possible to evoke natural sensations referred to the phantom limb. As part of the EU-funded TIME project, a computerized tool was developed for efficient sensory feedback evaluation in a multi-channel direct nerve stimulation system that may be used to provide more meaningful sensory feedback to amputee patients and consequently reduce PLP. Using sensory feedback to treat PLP or other chronic pain is still at an early stage of development. Multiple sensory modality feedback could also be considered as the focus of future work.

References

[1] L. Nikolajsen and T.S. Jensen. Phantom limb pain. *British Journal of Anaesthesia*, 87(1):107-116, 2001.

[2] P.A. Lacoux, I.K. Crombie, and W.A. Macrae. Pain in traumatic upper limb amputees in Sierra Leone. *Pain*, 99(1-2):309-312, 2002.

[3] P.L. Ephraim, S.T. Wegener, E.J. Mackenzie, T.R. Dillingham, and L.E. Pezzin. Phantom pain, residual limb pain, and back pain in amputees: Results of a national survey. *Archives of Physical Medicine and Rehabilitation*, 86(10):1910-1919, 2005.

[4] K. Ziegler-Graham, E.J. MacKenzie, P.L. Ephraim, T.G. Travison, and R.S. Brookmeyer. Estimating the Prevalence of Limb Loss in the United States: 2005 to 2050. *Archives of Physical Medicine and Rehabilitation*, 89(3):422-429, 2008.

[5] C.M. Kooijman, P.U. Dijkstra, J.H. B. Geertzen, A. Elzinga, and C.P. Van Der Schans. Phantom pain and phantom sensations in upper limb amputees: An epidemiological study. *Pain*, 87(1):33-41, 2000.

[6] S.M. Weinstein. Phantom limb pain and related disorders. *Neurologic Clinics*, 16(4):919-935, 1998.

[7] V.S. Ramachandran and W. Hirstein. The perception of phantom limbs. The D. O. Hebb lecture. *Brain*, 121(9):1603-1630, 1998.

[8] S.M. Grüsser et al. The relationship of perceptual phenomena and cortical reorganization in upper extremity amputees. *Neuroscience*, 102(2):263-272, 2001.

[9] V.S. Ramachandran, D.C. Rogers-Ramachandran, and S.K. Cobb. Touching the phantom limb. *Nature*, 377(6549):489-490, 1995.

[10] S.R. Weeks, V.C. Anderson-Barnes, and J.W. Tsao. Phantom limb pain: Theories and therapies. *Neurologist*, 16(5):277-286, 2010.

[11] E.J. Krane and L.B. Heller. The prevalence of phantom sensation and pain in pediatric amputees. *Journal of Pain and Symptom Management*, 10(1):21-29, 1995.

[12] R. Melzack, R. Israel, R. Lacroix, and G. Schultz. Phantom limbs in people with congenital limb deficiency or amputation in early childhood. *Brain*, 120(9):1603-1620, 1997.

[13] J.C. Bosmans, J.H. B. Geertzen, W.J. Post, C.P. Van Der Schans, and P.U. Dijkstra. Factors associated with phantom limb pain: A 3 1/2-year prospective study. *Clinical Rehabilitation*, 24(5):444-453, 2010.

[14] M.T. Schley et al. Painful and nonpainful phantom and stump sensations in acute traumatic amputees. *Journal of Trauma - Injury, Infection and Critical Care*, 65(4):858-864, 2008.

[15] C.M. Parkes. Factors determining the persistence of phantom pain in the amputee. *Journal of Psychosomatic Research*, 17(2):97-108, 1973.

[16] T.S. Jensen, B. Krebs, J.C. Nielsen, and P.C. Rasmussen. Phantom limb, phantom pain and stump pain in amputees during the first 6 months following limb amputation. *Pain*, 17(3):243-256, 1983.

[17] T.S. Jensen, B. Krebs, J.C. Nielsen, and P.C. Rasmussen. Immediate and long-term phantom limb pain in amputees: Incidence, clinical characteristics and relationship to pre-amputation limb pain. *Pain*, 21(3):267-278, 1985.

[18] L. Nikolajsen, S. Ilkjær, K. Króner, J.H. Christensen, and T.S. Jensen. The influence of preamputation pain on postamputation stump and phantom pain. *Pain*, 72(3):393-405, 1997.

[19] R. Melzack. Phantom limbs. *Scientific American*, 266(4):120-126, 1992.

[20] H. Flor et al. Phantom-limb pain as a perceptual correlate of cortical reorganization following arm amputation. *Nature*, 375(6531):482-484, 1995.

[21] S.W. Wartan, W.C. Hamann, J.R. Wedley, and I.M. McColl. Phantom pain and sensation among British veteran amputees. *British Journal of Anaesthesia*, 78(6):652-659, 1997.

[22] R.A. Sherman, C.J. Sherman, and I. Parker. Chronic phantom and stump pain among American veterans: Results of a survey. *Pain*, 18(1):83-95, 1984.

[23] A.P. Wolff et al. 21.Phantom pain. *Pain Practice*, 11(4):403-413, 2011.

[24] B. CRONHOLM. Phantom limbs in amputees; a study of changes in the integration of centripetal impulses with special reference to referred sensations. *Acta psychiatrica et neurologica Scandinavica. Supplementum*, 72:1-310, 1951.

[25] J.M. Katz. Psychophysiological contributions to phantom limbs. *Canadian Journal of Psychiatry*, 37(5):282-298, 1992.

[26] P. Montoya et al. The relationship of phantom limb pain to other phantom limb phenomena in upper extremity amputees. *Pain*, 72(1-2):87-93, 1997.

[27] R.A. Sherman, J.G. Arena, C.J. Sherman, and J.L. Ernst. The mystery of phantom pain: Growing evidence for psychophysiological mechanisms. *Biofeedback and Self-Regulation*, 14(4):267-280, 1989.

[28] J.G. Arena, A. Sherman, M. Bruno, and D. Smith. The relationship between situational stress and phantom limb pain: Cross-lagged correlational data from six month pain logs. *Journal of Psychosomatic Research*, 34(1):71-77, 1990.

[29] D. Richardson, M. Glenn, F. Horgan, and J. Nurmikko. A Prospective Study of Factors Associated With the Presence of Phantom Limb Pain Six Months After Major Lower Limb Amputation in Patients With Peripheral Vascular Disease. *Journal of Pain*, 8(10):793-801, 2007.

[30] A. Carabelli and C. Kellerman. Phantom limb pain: Relief by application of TENS to contralateral extremity. *Archives of Physical Medicine and Rehabilitation*, 66(7):466-467, 1985.

[31] S. Millstein, D. Bain, and A. Hunter. A review of employment patterns of industrial amputees: factors influencing rehabilitation. *Prosthetics and Orthotics International*, 9(2):69-78, 1985.

[32] E. pezzin, R. Dillingham, and J. Mackenzie. Rehabilitation and the long-term outcomes of persons with trauma-related amputations. *Archives of Physical Medicine and Rehabilitation*, 81(3):292-300, 2000.

[33] D.M. Ehde et al. Chronic phantom sensations, phantom pain, residual limb pain, and other regional pain after lower limb amputation. *Archives of Physical Medicine and Rehabilitation*, 81(8):1039-1044, 2000.

[34] A. Hanley, D.M. Ehde, M. Campbell, O. Osborn, and G. Smith. Self-reported treatments used for lower-limb phantom pain: Descriptive findings. *Archives of Physical Medicine and Rehabilitation*, 87(2):270-277, 2006.

[35] H. Flor. Phantom-limb pain: Characteristics, causes, and treatment. *Lancet Neurology*, 1(3):182-189, 2002.

[36] M. Costigan, J. Scholz, and J. Woolf. Neuropathic pain: A maladaptive response of the nervous system to damage. *Annual Review of Neuroscience*, 32:1-32, June 2009.

[37] X. Navarro, M. Vivó, and A. Valero-Cabré. Neural plasticity after peripheral nerve injury and regeneration. *Progress in Neurobiology*, 82(4):163-201, 2007.

[38] G. Di Pino, E. Guglielmelli, and M. Rossini. Neuroplasticity in amputees: Main implications on bidirectional interfacing of cybernetic hand prostheses. *Progress in Neurobiology*, 88(2):114-126, 2009.

[39] G. Devor, R. Govrin-Lippmann, and J. Angelides. Na+ channel immunolocalization in peripheral mammalian axons and changes following nerve injury and neuroma formation. *Journal of Neuroscience*, 13(5):1976-1992, 1993.

[40] G. Devor, W. Jänig, and M. Michaelis. Modulation of activity in dorsal root ganglion neurons by sympathetic activation in nerve-injured rats. *Journal of Neurophysiology*, 71(1):38-47, 1994.

[41] A. Sherman and C.J. Sherman. Prevalence and characteristics of chronic phantom limb pain among American veterans. Results of a trial survey. *American Journal of Physical Medicine*, 62(5):227-238, 1983.

[42] L. Carlen, D. Wall, H. Nadvorna, and T.V. Steinbach. Phantom limbs and related phenomena in recent traumatic amputations. *Neurology*, 28(3):211-217, 1978.

[43] R. Baron. Mechanisms of disease: Neuropathic pain - A clinical perspective. *Nature Clinical Practice Neurology*, 2(2):95-106, 2006.

[44] H. Flor, L. Nikolajsen, and S. Jensen. Phantom limb pain: A case of maladaptive CNS plasticity. *Nature Reviews Neuroscience*, 7(11):873-881, 2006.

[45] S. Ramachandran, C. Rogers-Ramachandran, G. Stewart, and T.P. Pons. Perceptual correlates of massive cortical reorganization. *Science*, 258(5085):1159-1160, 1992.

[46] E.J. Hall, D. Flament, C.M. Fraser, and R.N. Lemon. Non-invasive brain stimulation reveals reorganised cortical outputs in amputees. *Neuroscience Letters*, 116(3):379-386, 1990.

[47] R. Chen, L.G. Cohen, and M. Hallett. Nervous system reorganization following injury. *Neuroscience*, 111(4,6):761-773, 2002.

[48] T.R. Elbert et al. Extensive reorganization of the somatosensory cortex in adult humans after nervous system injury. *NeuroReport*, 5(18):2593-2597, 1994.

[49] T.T. Yang et al. Sensory maps in the human brain. *Nature*, 368(6472):592-593, 1994.

[50] M. Lotze, H. Flor, W. Grodd, W. Larbig, and N.P. Birbaumer. Phantom movements and pain an fMRI study in upper limb amputees. *Brain*, 124(11):2268-2277, 2001.

[51] A. Karl, N.P. Birbaumer, W. Lutzenberger, L.G. Cohen, and H. Flor. Reorganization of motor and somatosensory cortex in upper extremity amputees with phantom limb pain. *Journal of Neuroscience*, 21(10):3609-3618, 2001.

[52] A. Karl, W. Mühlnickel, R. Kurth, and H. Flor. Neuroelectric source imaging of steady-state movement-related cortical potentials in human upper extremity amputees with and without phantom limb pain. *Pain*, 110(1-2):90-102, 2004.

[53] S.L. Florence, T.A. Hackett, and F. Strata. Thalamic and cortical contributions to neural plasticity after limb amputation. *Journal of Neurophysiology*, 83(5):3154-3159, 2000.

[54] M. Diers, C. Christmann, C. Koeppe, M. Ruf, and H. Flor. Mirrored, imagined and executed movements differentially activate sensorimotor cortex in amputees with and without phantom limb pain. *Pain*, 149(2):296-304, 2010.

[55] K.D. Davis et al. Phantom sensations generated by thalamic microstimulation. *Nature*, 391(6665):385-387, 1998.

[56] S.L. Florence and J.H. Kaas. Large-scale reorganization at multiple levels of the somatosensory pathway follows therapeutic amputation of the hand in monkeys. *Journal of Neuroscience*, 15(12):8083-8095, 1995.

[57] E.R. Ergenzinger, M.M. Glasier, J.O. Hahm, and T.P. Pons. Cortically induced thalamic plasticity in the primate somatosensory system. *Nature Neuroscience*, 1(3):226-229, 1998.

[58] J. Alviar, T. Hale, and M. Dungca. Pharmacologic interventions for treating phantom limb pain. *Cochrane database of systematic reviews (Online)*, 12:CD006380, 2011.

[59] R.G. Bittar, S. Otero, H.R.. Carter, and T.Z. Aziz. Deep brain stimulation for phantom limb pain. *Journal of Clinical Neuroscience*, 12(4):399-404, 2005.

[60] N.J. Ray et al. Abnormal thalamocortical dynamics may be altered by deep brain stimulation: Using magnetoencephalography to study phantom limb pain. *Journal of Clinical Neuroscience*, 16(1):32-36, 2009.

[61] Y. Katayama et al. Motor cortex stimulation for phantom limb pain: Comprehensive therapy with spinal cord and thalamic stimulation. *Stereotactic and Functional Neurosurgery*, 77(1-4):159-162, 2002.

[62] J.C. Sol et al. Chronic motor cortex stimulation for phantom limb pain: Correlations between pain relief and functional imaging studies. *Stereotactic and Functional Neurosurgery*, 77(1-4):172-176, 2002.

[63] M. Gehling and M. Tryba. Prophylaxis of phantom pain: Is regional analgesia ineffective? *Schmerz*, 17(1):11-19, 2003.

[64] A.W. Lambert et al. Randomized prospective study comparing preoperative epidural and intraoperative perineural analgesia for the prevention of postoperative stump and phantom limb pain following major amputation. *Regional Anesthesia and Pain Medicine*, 26(4):316-321, 2001.

[65] G. Belleggia and N.P. Birbaumer. Treatment of phantom limb pain with combined EMG and thermal biofeedback: A case report. *Applied Psychophysiology Biofeedback*, 26(2):141-146, 2001.

[66] R.A. Sherman, N.G. Gall, and J. Gormly. Treatment of phantom limb pain with muscular relaxation training to disrupt the pain-anxiety-tension cycle. *Pain*, 6(1):47-55, 1979.

[67] N. Harden et al. Biofeedback in the treatment of phantom limb pain: A time-series analysis. *Applied Psychophysiology Biofeedback*, 30(1):83-93, 2005.

[68] R. Chan. Hypnosis and phantom limb pain. *Australian Journal of Clinical and Experimental Hypnosis*, 34(1):55-64, 2006.

[69] L.M. Black, R.K. Persons, and B. Jamieson. What is the best way to manage phantom limb pain? *Journal of Family Practice*, 58(3):155-158, 2009.

[70] J.A. Halbert, M. Crotty, and I.D. Cameron. Evidence for the optimal management of acute and chronic phantom pain: A systematic review. *Clinical Journal of Pain*, 18(2):84-92, 2002.

[71] R.A. Sherman. Postamputation pain. In *Clinical Pain Management: Chronic Pain*, T.S. Jensen, P.R. Wilson, and A.S. Rice (Eds.). London, Hodder Arnold Publishing, 2002, ch. 32:427-436.

[72] V.S. Ramachandran and D. Rodgers-Ramachandran. Synaesthesia in phantom limbs induced with mirrors. *Proceedings of the Royal Society B: Biological Sciences*, 263(1369):377-386, 1996.

[73] B.L. Chan et al. Mirror therapy for phantom limb pain. *New England Journal of Medicine*, 357(21):2206-2207, 2007.

[74] T. Lundeberg. Relief of pain from a phantom limb by peripheral stimulation. *Journal of Neurology*, 232(2):79-82, 1985.

[75] S.M. Mannix, C. O'Sullivan, and G.A. Kelly. Acupuncture for managing phantom-limb syndrome: A systematic review. *Medical Acupuncture*, 25(1):23-42, 2013.

[76] K. MacIver, D. Lloyd, S.A. Kelly, N.J. Roberts, and T.J. Nurmikko. Phantom limb pain, cortical reorganization and the therapeutic effect of mental imagery. *Brain*, 131(8):2181-2191, 2008.

[77] K.G. Rasmussen and T.A. Rummans. Electroconvulsive therapy for phantom limb pain. *Pain*, 85(1-2):297-299, 2000.

[78] C.Y. Huang, R. Yang, T. Kuo, and K.H. Hsu. Phantom limb pain treated by far infrared ray. In *Proceedings of the 31st Annual International Conference of the IEEE Engineering in Medicine and Biology Society: Engineering the Future of Biomedicine, EMBC 2009*, Minneapolis, 2009:1589-1591.

[79] I. Bókkon, A. Till, F. Grass, and A. Erdöfi Szabó. Phantom pain reduction by low-frequency and low-intensity electromagnetic fields. *Electromagnetic Biology and Medicine*, 30(3):115-127, 2011.

[80] W.M. Jenkins, M.M. Merzenich, M.T. Ochs, T.T. Allard, and E. Guic-Robles. Functional reorganization of primary somatosensory cortex in adult owl monekys after behaviorally controlled tactile stimulation. *Journal of Neurophysiology*, 63(1):82-104, 1990.

[81] G.H. Recanzone, M.M. Merzenich, W.M. Jenkins, K.A. Grajski, and H.R. Dinse. Topographic reorganization of the hand representation in cortical area 3b of owl monkeys trained in a frequency-discrimination task. *Journal of Neurophysiology*, 67(5):1031-1056, 1992.

[82] S. Knecht et al. Reorganizational and perceptional changes after amputation. *Brain*, 119(4):1213-1219, 1996.

[83] H. Flor. The modification of cortical reorganization and chronic pain by sensory feedback. *Applied Psychophysiology Biofeedback*, 27(3):215-227, 2002.

[84] H. Flor, C. Denke, M.J. Schaefer, and S.M. Grüsser. Effect of sensory discrimination training on cortical reorganisation and phantom limb pain. *Lancet*, 357(9270):1763-1764, 2001.

[85] M. Lotze et al. Does use of a myoelectric prosthesis prevent cortical reorganization and phantom limb pain? *Nature Neuroscience*, 2(6):501-502, 1999.

[86] P.M. Rossini et al. Double nerve intraneural interface implant on a human amputee for robotic hand control. *Clinical Neurophysiology*, 121(5):777-783, 2010.

[87] C. Dietrich et al. Sensory feedback prosthesis reduces phantom limb pain: Proof of a principle. *Neuroscience Letters*, 507(2):97-100, 2012.

[88] L. Moseley, N.M. Zalucki, and K. Wiech. Tactile discrimination, but not tactile stimulation alone, reduces chronic limb pain. *Pain*, 137(3):600-608, 2008.

[89] K.A. Kaczmarek, J.G. Webster, P. Bach-y-Rita, and W.J. Tompkins. Electrotactile and vibrotactile displays for sensory substitution systems. *IEEE Transactions on Biomedical Engineering*, 38(1):1-16, 1991.

[90] G. F. Shannon. A comparison of alternative means of providing sensory feedback on upper limb prostheses. *Medical and Biology Engineering*, 14(3):289-294, 1976.

[91] A.P. Toney, L.E. Dunne, B.H. Thomas, and S.P. Ashdown. A shoulder pad insert vibrotactile display. In *Proceedings - International Symposium on Wearable Computers, ISWC*, White Plains, NY, United States, 2003:35-44.

[92] C. Pylatiuk, A. Kargov, and S.M. Schulz. Design and evaluation of a low-cost force feedback system for myoelectric prosthetic hands. *Journal of Prosthetics and Orthotics*, 18(2):57-61, 2006.

[93] H. Witteveen, J.S. Rietman, and P. Veltink. Grasping force and slip feedback through vibrotactile stimulation to be used in myoelectric forearm prostheses. In *Proceedings of the Annual International Conference of the IEEE Engineering in Medicine and Biology Society, EMBS*, San Diego, CA, United States, 2012:2969-2972.

[94] A.Y. szeto and F.A. Saunders. Electrocutaneous stimulation for sensory communication in rehabilitation engineering. *IEEE Transactions on Biomedical Engineering*, BME-29(4):300-308, 1982.

[95] E.A. Pfeiffer. Electrical stimulation of sensory nerves with skin electrodes for research, diagnosis, communication and behavioral conditioning: A survey. *Medical & Biological Engineering*, 6(6):637-651, 1968.

[96] R.N. Scott, R.R. Caldwell, R.H. Brittain, A.B. Cameron, and V.A. Dunfield. Sensory-feedback system compatible with myoelectric control. *Medical & Biological Engineering and Computing*, 18(1):65-69, 1980.

[97] R.E. Prior, J.H. Lyman, P.A. Case, and C.M. Scott. Supplemental sensory feedback for the VA/NU myoelectric hand. Background and preliminary designs. *Bulletin of Prosthetics Research*, 10(26):170-191, 1976.

[98] G.F. Shannon. A myoelectrically-controlled prosthesis with sensory feedback. *Medical & Biological Engineering and Computing*, 17(1):73-80, 1979.

[99] H. Schmidl. The importance of information feedback in prostheses for the upper limbs. *Prosthetics and Orthotics International*, 1(1):21-24, 1977.

[100] T.W. Beeker, J. During, and A. Den Hertog. Artificial touch in a hand-prosthesis. *Medical & biological engineering*, 5(1):47-49, 1967.

[101] G.S. Dhillon, T.B. Krüger, J.S. Sandhu, and K.W. Horch. Effects of short-term training on sensory and motor function in severed nerves of long-term human amputees. *Journal of Neurophysiology*, 93(5):2625-2633, 2005.

[102] G.A. Gescheider. *Psychophysics: The Fundamentals*. 3rd ed.Mahwah, NJ, Lawrence Erlbaum Associates, 1997.

[103] W.H. Ehrenstein and A. Ehrenstein. Psychophysical methods. In *Modern Techniques in Neuroscience Research*, U. Windhorst and H. Johansson (Eds.). Berlin, Springer, 1999, ch. 43:1211-1241.

[104] S.S. Stevens. On the psychophysical law. *Psychological Review*, 64(3):153-181, 1957.

[105] S.J. Grant et al. A comparison of the reproducibility and the sensitivity to change of visual analogue scales , Borg scales, and likert scales in normal subjects during submaximal exercise. *Chest*, 116(5):1208-1217, 1999.

[106] T. Boretius et al. A transverse intrafascicular multichannel electrode (TIME) to interface with the peripheral nerve. *Biosensors and Bioelectronics*, 26(1):62-69, 2010.

[107] J.P. Girvin et al. Electrocutaneous stimulation I. The effects of stimulus parameters on absolute threshold. *Perception and Psychophysics*, 32(6):524-528, 1982.

[108] G. Kantor, G. Alon, and H. Ho. The effects of selected stimulus waveforms on pulse and phase characteristics at sensory and motor thresholds. *Physical Therapy*, 74(10):951-962, 1994.

[109] S.T. Palmer, D.J. Martin, W.M. Steedman, and J. Ravey. Alteration of interferential current and transcutaneous electrical nerve stimulation frequency: Effects on nerve excitation. *Archives of Physical Medicine and Rehabilitation*, 80(9):1065-1071, 1999.

[110] J. Chae and R.L. Hart. Comparison of discomfort associated with surface and percutaneous intramuscular electrical stimulation for persons with chronic hemiplegia. *American Journal of Physical Medicine and Rehabilitation*, 77(6):516-522, 1998.

[111] R.K. Garnsworthy, R.L. Gully, P. Kenins, and R.A. Westerman. ranscutaneous electrical stimulation and the sensation of prickle. *Journal of Neurophysiology*, 59(4):1116-1127, 1988.

[112] A. Kuhn, T. Keller, M.F. Lawrence, and M. Morari. The influence of electrode size on selectivity and comfort in transcutaneous electrical stimulation of the forearm. *IEEE Transactions on Neural Systems and Rehabilitation Engineering*, 18(3):255-262, 2010.

[113] S.C. Naaman, R.B. Stein, and C. Thomas. Minimizing discomfort with surface neuromuscular stimulation. *Neurorehabilitation and Neural Repair*, 14(3):223-228, 2000.

[114] F. Gračanin and A. Trnkoczy. Optimal stimulus parameters for minimum pain in the chronic stimulation of innervated muscle. *Archives of Physical Medicine and Rehabilitation*, 56(6):243-249, 1975.

[115] E.M. Van Der Heide, J.R. Buitenweg, E. Marani, and W.L. C. Rutten. Single pulse and pulse train modulation of cutaneous electrical stimulation: A comparison of methods. *Journal of Clinical Neurophysiology*, 26(1):54-60, 2009.

[116] R.M. Sachs, J.D. Miller, and K.W. Grant. Perceived magnitude of multiple electrocutaneous pulses. *Perception & Psychophysics*, 28(3):255-262, 1980.

[117] G.S. Dhillon and K.W. Horch. Direct neural sensory feedback and control of a prosthetic arm. *IEEE Transactions on Neural Systems and Rehabilitation Engineering*, 13(4):468-472, 2005.

[118] A.Y. Szeto, J.H. Lyman, and R.E. Prior. Electrocutaneous pulse rate and pulse width psychometric functions for sensory communications. *Human Factors*, 21(2):241-249, 1979.

[119] N.P. Birbaumer. Effects of regional anesthesia on phantom limb pain are mirrored in changes in cortical reorganization. *Journal of Neuroscience*, 17(14):5503-5508, 1997.

[120] C.M. Michel et al. EEG source imaging. *Clinical Neurophysiology*, 115(10):2195-2222, 2004.

About the author

Bo Geng was born in 1979 in Shanxi, China. She received the M.Sc. degree in electrical engineering from Institute of Electronics, Chinese Academy of Sciences, Beijing, China in 2005, and Ph.D. degree in biomedical engineering and science from Aalborg University, Aalborg, Denmark in 2013. During 2009-2010, she was a visiting scholar in the Biomedical Department at IUPUI, Indianapolis in the United States. She was awarded an Elite Research Scholarship and Chinese Government Scholarship for Outstanding Self-Financed Students Abroad in 2010 and 2011, respectively. Her research interests include artificial sensory feedback, sensory substitution, sensory augmentation, phantom limb pain treatment and mechanisms, and use of electrical stimulation in neurorehabilitation.